THE COMPLETE

AIR FRYER COOKBOOK

FOR BEGINNERS:

EASY, DELICIOUS AND BUDGET FRIENDLY AIR FRYER RECIPES FOR HEALTHY LIVING

By

Bobby Chef & Emily Cook

Disclaimer

The information provided in this book is designed to provide helpful
information on the subjects discussed. The publisher and author are not
responsible for any specific health or allergy needs that may require medical
supervision and are not liable for any damages or negative consequences from
any treatment, action, application or preparation, to any person reading or
following the information in this book.

Table of Contents

INTRODUCTION

The influence of technology has had a remarkable effect on every aspect of human life and this includes cooking. Air frying is a modern method of grilling, frying, baking and roasting without the use of a copious amount of oil, yet providing a deep-fried taste and texture.

The traditional frying method often requires that you submerge your food in hot oil, but, with the use of Hot air frying machines, your food ends up crispy on the outside and very moist on the inside without the use of such amount of oil. I would like to believe that the air fryer a fantastic kitchen innovation, and probably one of the best kitchen appliances since microwaves and slow cookers came into existence.

The air-fryer is designed to circulate extremely hot air in a fashion that mimics the movement and flow of heat currents in a pot of boiling oil, to crisp up the outsides of food while cooking it on the inside. Some designs also have a grilling element, for added browning and crispiness.

WHAT IS AN AIR FRYER?

An air fryer is a kitchen appliance used for frying, grilling, and roasting. In other words, it is an appliance meant for cooking meals like potato chips, chicken, fish, and so many other forms of food that requires frying roasting or grilling. The air fryer makes use of what is called a mechanical fan, this fan is inbuilt into the fryer, the mechanical fan circulates the hot air around the food at high speed, and in-turn cooking the food in such a way that a crispy texture is formed and the interior of the meal becomes well cooked.

Air fryers are very healthy devices for cooking; the methods used by these appliances are different from the traditional methods of frying. The circulating hot air in the pot does the cooking thereby reducing the quantity of fat in the food and leaving no room for calories that may, in turn, become hazardous to human health, thus cooking becomes more healthy, safe and efficiently. The air fryer is also economical; as it reduces the cost of cooking, in other words, less amount of money is spent on buying oil.

The air fryer is safe for cooking, but it is important that you have a basic knowledge of how the air fryer works. Firstly, the fryer has two major openings, one at the top and the other at the back. The opening at the top is meant for taking air into the fryer while the exhaust at the back is meant to control the temperature in the fryer by releasing any undesired hot air it is also used to control an increase in internal pressure.

Air fryers are often programmed differently; it depends on the producers of the fryer. The temperature inside a fryer can go up to 200°C/400°F; it depends on the model and the company. Due to the nature of the hot air, it is as safer not to put oil or all other inflammable either inside or near the fryer.

A popularly known company that produces air fryers is the go wise industry. The air fryers from this company are of top quality, they more evenly, effectively and faster. However, some of the descriptions in this cookbook conform to the methods used in operating the power Air fryer XL model. I recommend you know how your fryer work, so you can change the instructions to suit your fryer.

BENEFITS OF AIR FRYERS

The benefits of using air fryers cannot be overemphasized, but for knowledge sakes, the air fryer is one of the best appliances used for cooking specific forms of food that requires frying, roasting or grilling without the without the use of excess oil. It is only essential that you brush your meal with a little oil so as to prevent it from sticking to the surfaces of the pan. But this is only required when using some certain types of fryers, when using expensive air fryers, you may not have any brushing to do. The following are the benefits of the air fryer

ECONOMIC BENEFITS:

Around 80 to 90% less oil is used for frying when using air fryers. When compared to the traditional gas fryer and other forms of frying, that is a lot of cost reduction. In cases where you may need to use oil, the quantity of oil you may need for brushing your food may be little.

HEALTH BENEFITS:

A very small amount of oil is required for brushing the food before keeping it inside the air fryer; this means that air fryers are more beneficial than other forms of frying.

Similarly, the air fryer comes along with an air filter; this helps to ensure that the air released through the fryer is always clean.

ENERGY CONSERVATION:

Air fryers consume less electronic energy than conventional, electronic cooking appliances like deep fryers etc. A subtle amount of heat is generated inside the air fryer; this heat moves freely all over a smaller space, and the heat is well distributed evenly.

Most importantly for me, the fragrance generated when you cook food in an air fryer, it creates no similar prolonged smell which usually a conventional oven doesn't.

SAFETY BENEFITS:

Hot oil burns are a common cause of hospital admission in the United Kingdom; similarly, it estimated that about 2,600 fire out brakes in the United Kingdom on a yearly basis is as a result of deep fat frying. In the United States, it is known to have caused 1,230 non-fatal casualties and 12 fatalities, from 2008 to 2010. There is an estimated average of 164,500 household fires out brake in a year, and 51% of those are caused by cooking with oil, fat or grease. Hot air frying tremendously reduces the danger of possible accidents that could occur out of making fried food. Things become extremely easier when young teenagers, adults and the elderly can be taught to fry with less fear of cooking hazards or any safety concerns.

HOW TO USE AN AIR FRYER

Using the fryer is quite cool and easy to learn, the following are a few tips or basics, you should know.

1. COOKING TEMPERATURE:

Depending on the sort of food you intend to fry or grill, the required temperature may differ. It is only important that you take note of the required heat level need to get your food well cooked, if you will need to deep fry in oil at 325°F, you will still need to set your air fryer to cook at that same level. The same rule applies when it comes to roasting. This adjustment is needed because the circulating air makes the heat of the cooking environment more consistent, and thus more intense than traditional cooking instructions. Similarly, it is important that the air fryer is preheated before putting any food in it. Use your menu to determine the appropriate heat level for preheating your appliances.

2. TOSS COOKING ITEMS WITH OIL, SPARINGLY:

It is important that you prepare the fryer before using it, this will help you get efficient results, firstly, fatty foods chicken, meatballs etc. Do not need to be tossed with any form of oil. When cooking nonfatty foods like plantain and potatoes, the food should be sprayed with at least two tablespoons of oil before it is placed in the basket. This will help to give your food a golden brown and crispy taste

Similarly, a cooking spray should be used on the air fryer basket or on the rack before putting sticky foods that are already coated or battered in flour.

THE FROZEN FOODS EXCEPTION:

Frozen and par-cooked foods, such as fish sticks and chicken strips, can usually be air-fried without any form of oil, but it is recommended that you spray the fryer basket or racks to prevent any sticking

3. FILL THE AIR FRYER BASKET OR RACK:

It is not advisable to stack up floured and battered food when air frying, this can be done if the model allows for such, but in order to get best cooking results, I will advise that you cook your meal in sets. Similarly, you should as well try to shake up your food every 3-5 minutes so as to get an evenly cooked meal.

4. CHECK FOR DONENESS EARLY:
In general, we have explained that the air fryer is a very good cooking appliance, but that requires proper management. While cooking is been done, it is advisable that you occasionally check the meal, so as to keep yourself acquainted with the texture you may want to get from the food.

THE DIFFERENCES BETWEEN AIR FRYING AND DEEP-FAT FRYING

TASTE

If the modes of cooking are different, then so should the taste of the meal, the decisions on preferred options are often dependent on individuals preferences. Yet, the taste is acceptably close to that of the deep-fried. The most important part is that the quantity of calorie consumed is far less than what is obtainable with deep frying. With the use of the air fryer, frying has become way easier than you used to know.

TIMING

Air fryer takes far more cooking time than the traditional frying instructions, for example, when making deep fries, it takes 25 minutes on the air fryer and 8 minutes on the deep fryer. Hot air frying completely eliminates all the hassle of cleaning, frying, and oiling.

HEALTH BENEFITS

With the use of hot air fryers, your favorite foods are back on the menu, and dieticians will definitely not object. For individuals with health complications like diabetes and high blood pressure etc. Eating oily food may not be recommended. Air frying has greatly put a limit to this and the most interesting thing about air frying is that it allows you to use healthy oil like walnut oil, avocado oil, grape-seed oil, etc. For your frying with having to send much in buying these forms oil in large quantity.

AVAILABLE AIR FRYER BRANDS/MODELS TO PICK FROM

1. PHILIPS XL AIR FRYER

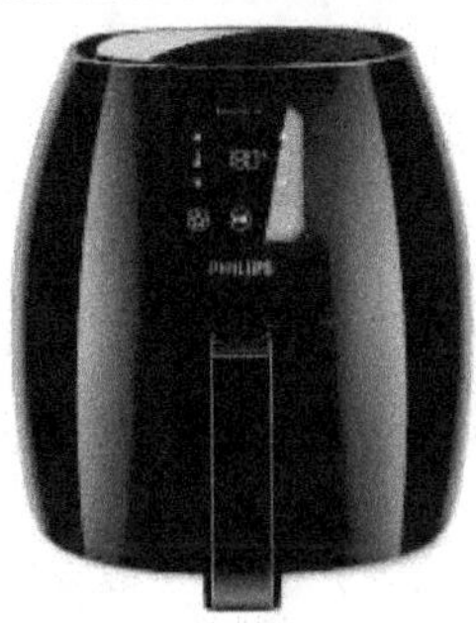

Features

1) Safe and easy to clean

2) Highly efficient air frying technology

3) A digital touchscreen interface

4) Heat adjustment of up to 360 degrees Celsius

5) 60-minute timer with ready signal and auto shut-off

6) Smart preset button

2. T-FAL FZ7002 ACTIFRY

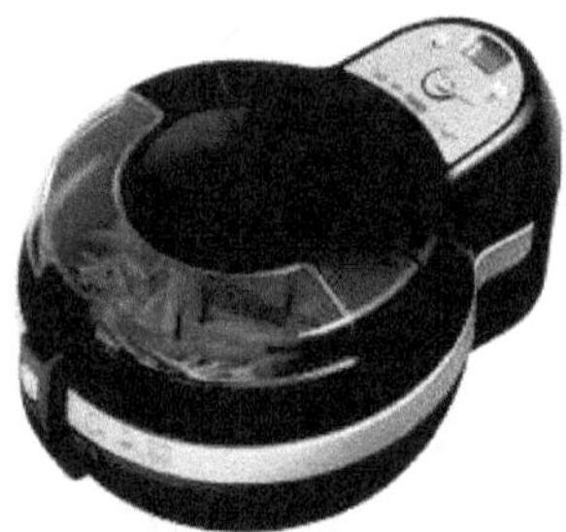

Features

1) Simple on/off switch

2) digital countdown timer with buzzer for easy monitoring

3) Removable ceramic-coated nonstick pan

4) Secure lid for safe splatter-free cooking

5) stay-cool exterior; a filter for odorless cooking

6) Free 38 recipe book and measuring spoon included;

7) Dishwasher-safe parts for quick cleanup

3. Gowise USA GW22621

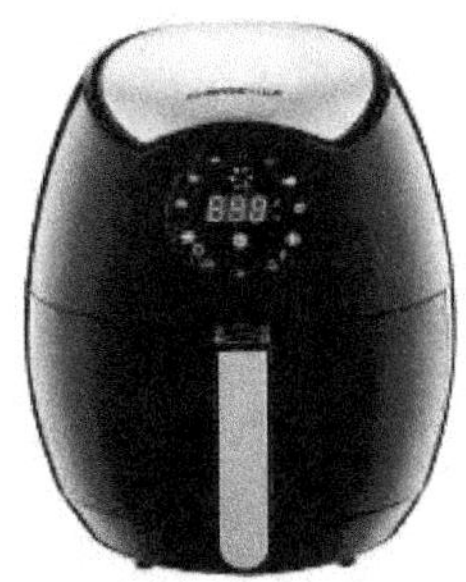

Features:

1. These appliances have multiple cooking presets to make cooking more easy and healthy.
2. LCD display
3. Multiple cooking menus.
4. Go wise air fryers have rapid air circulation system installed within it.
5. Automatic standby mode and safety features are provided with these go wise air fryers.

4. Avalon Bay Digital Air Fryer

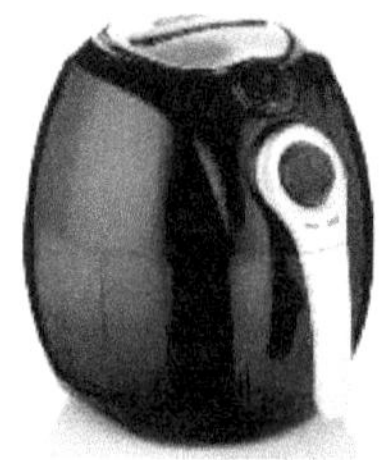

Features:

1) 3.7 Quart capacity, temperatures ranging from 180 to 400 Degrees,

2) Non-slip feet, 30-minute timer,

3) 1400 watts of power,

4) Non-BPA plastic and a detachable basket for easy food transfer.

5) A non-stick baking dish,

6) Multi-use rack.

AIR FRYER BREAKFAST RECIPES

Air-fryer Baked Eggs in Bread Bowls

COOKING ITEMS:

Crusty dinner rolls (use 4 pieces or as many as you want)

4 pieces of eggs (large eggs are better)

Chopped and mixed parsley, chives, tarragon leaves (4 tablespoons)

Heavy cream (use 4 tablespoons)

Grated parmesan cheese

Salt

Pepper

INSTRUCTIONS:

1) Slice off the top of a dinner roll and preserve in a clean bowl, carefully pinch out the dinner rolls till you make a hole that can comfortably accommodate a single egg.

2) Separately crack an egg into a small clean bowl, one egg for each dinner roll. Before purring the egg into each dinner roll, top each egg with some herbs and a bit of cream. Season with salt and pepper. Sprinkle with Parmesan and pour into the dinner rolls.

3) Preheat the air fryer

4) Put the dinner rolls into the air fryer and set the fryer to bake at a 350°F (180°C) for 20-25 minutes, until the bread is toasted and set aside

5) After 20 minutes, place the preserved bread tops on a baking sheet and bake until golden brown. Let it sit for 5 minutes and place the tops on the roll

6) Serve warm and enjoy.

Air-fryer Breakfast soufflé

COOKING ITEMS:

4 pieces of eggs

Light cream (use 4 tablespoons)

Red chili pepper

Fresh Parsley leaf (finely chopped)

INSTRUCTIONS:

1) Break the egg into a bowl, stir in the cream, chopped parsley, the red chili pepper and stir

2) Fill the soufflé cups halfway with the egg mixture.

3) Preheat the air fryer

4) Set the fryer to heat up at 392°F (200°C) and let the dishes sit in the fryer for 8 minutes, but if you want soufflés baveux soft, then a 5 minutes cooking is enough.

Potatoes Au Gratin

COOKING ITEMS

Russet potatoes (use 7 medium pieces, but peel them before use)

Milk (use ½ a cup)

Cream (use ½ a cup)

Black pepper (use 1 teaspoon)

½ teaspoon of Nutmeg

½ cup of semi-mature cheese (to be grated)

INSTRUCTIONS:

1) Preheat the Air Fryer at 390°F

2) Make thin slices of the potatoes

3) Mix ½ cup of milk and ½ cup of cream in a clean bowl, season with salt, pepper, and nutmeg to taste

4) Coat the potato slices with the milk mixture.

5) Place the coated potato slices into an 8-inch heat resistant baking dish and pour the remaining mixture on top

6) Place the baking dish in the cooking basket and put the basket into the Air Fryer.

7) Set the fryer to cook at 390°F for 25 minutes.

8) Open the fryer, remove the basket, and distribute the cheese evenly over the potatoes.

9) Place the basket back into the fryer and let the fryer cook for another 10 minutes and bake the gratin until it is nicely browned.

Breakfast Burrito Recipe

COOKING ITEMS

3-4 Slices of Turkey or Chicken Breast

2 pieces of Eggs (large eggs are better)

1/4 Red Bell Pepper, to be Sliced

1/4 Avocado, to be Sliced

1/8 Cup of Grated Mozzarella Cheese

2 Tablespoons of Salsa

Pinch of Salt

Pepper

Tortilla

INSTRUCTIONS:

1) Break the two eggs into a small bowl, and pinch of salt and pepper as desired, and beat it till its smooth.

2) Preheat the fryer to 200°C for up to 5 minutes,

3) Pour the egg mixture into a small shallow non-stick pan and place the pan in the Air fryer basket. Cook the egg in the Air fryer at 200°C for 5 minutes.

4) After 5 minutes, open the fryer and remove the pan from the basket and set aside.

5) Start filling your tortilla with the egg, chicken breast, red pepper, avocado, cheese, and salsa. Carefully and loosely wrap it up.

6) Open the fryer and place the burrito into the basket. Set the fryer to Heat up the burrito in the Air fryer at 180°C for 3 minutes to 5 minutes.

7) Dish with salsa

8) Serve and enjoy!

Air-fryer Easy Breakfast Sandwich

COOKING ITEMS:

Range egg (use 1 piece)

English bacon (use 1 piece)

English muffin (use 1 piece)

A pinch of salt

Pepper to taste

INSTRUCTIONS:

1) Crack the egg into a clean bowl; add salt and pepper to taste and pour it into an ovenproof soufflé cup.

2) Preheat the air fryer

3) Place the egg, bacon, and muffin into the air-fryer.

4) Turn the air-fryer to heat up at 200°C for 4 -6 minutes.

5) Assemble the sandwich

6) Serve and enjoy

Air Fryer Greasy Home Fried Potatoes

COOKING ITEMS

Potatoes (use 3 large pieces, wash and dice into smaller chunks)

Onion (use 1 piece, to be sliced and diced)

Small Red Pepper (use i-2 pieces, slice, and dice)

2-3 Tablespoons of coconut oil (gee or bacon Greece will do)

1-2 tbsp. Of Sea Salt

Powdered onion (use 1 teaspoon)

Powder garlic (use 1 teaspoon)

Paprika (use 1 teaspoon)

INSTRUCTIONS

1) Slice the potatoes and place into a bowl of water and soak for 20 minutes.

2) Mix together all seasonings in a separate clean bowl and set aside.

3) Grease the bottom of your Air Fryer Basket with Coconut Oil or whichever form of oil you have.

4) Preheat the fryer

5) Drain to soaked potatoes, add 2 tablespoons of oils and mix.

6) Place the potatoes into Air Fryer Basket.

7) Cook potatoes in the fryer at for 20 minutes at 200° C,

8) Periodically check the sliced potatoes and shake several times to ensure even cooking.

9) Dice onions and red peppers into mixing bowl, add seasoning and set aside.

10) Transfer the cooked potatoes to a bowl with onions and peppers and mix through.

11) Put mixture into Air Fryer Basket and place into the Air Fryer.

12) Allow fryer to cook 200°C for 5-10 more minutes

13) Turn off the fryer, remove the basket then dish and serve

Spanish Frittata with Potato and Chorizo

COOKING ITEMS

Jumbo free range eggs (3 pieces)

Half chorizo sausage (to be sliced)

1 big potato (par-boiled and cubed)

Frozen corn (use half a cup)

Olive oil

Chopped fresh parsley leaf (or use any other herbs of your choice)

Wheel of feta

Salt

Pepper

Tomato relish

Fresh rockets

INSTRUCTIONS:

1) Pour a little oil into the nonstick pan; place on stove, add chorizo, corn and the potato and let it steam for a while

2) Preheat the air fryer

3) Set the Air Fryer to cook at 180°C.

4) Place the sausage and potato into the basket and cook until slightly browned and set aside (periodically check if brown)

5) Break the 3 eggs into a clean bowl, garnish with seasoning and beat until smooth

6) Pour eggs over the potato and sausage in and top with crumbled feta and chopped fresh parsley (or any other herb).

7) Cook in the fryer for another 5 to 10 minutes at 180°C,

8) When cooked, serve garnished with a chunky tomato relish and some fresh rocket.

Air-fryer Easy Full English

COOKING ITEMS:

Chestnut mushrooms (8 pieces)

Tomatoes (use 8 pieces, slice each potato in two)

A clove of garlic, (minced or crushed)

4 rashers of smoked back bacon

Chipolatas (use for pieces)

Baby leaf spinach (200 grams)

Eggs (4 pieces)

INSTRUCTIONS:

1. Preheat the air-fryer to 200°C.

2. Spray a tin that could fit into the fryer basket and Put in the mushrooms, tomatoes, and garlic into the round tin.

3. Place the tin, bacon and chipolatas basket and place into the fryer; and let it cook for 10 minutes.

4. Pour hot water into the baby spinach and drain well.

5. Bring out tin from the fryer, spray in the spinach and crack in the eggs.

6. Reduce the temperature to 160°C and cook for another 5 minutes

Apricot Blackberry Crumble

COOKING ITEMS:

Fresh apricots (use 18 ounces)

Fresh blackberries (5½ ounces)

½ cup sugar

Lemon juice (2 teaspoons)

White flour (1 cup)

Salt

Butter (5 tablespoons)

INSTRUCTIONS:

1. Remove the stones from the apricots and cut them into cubes, then place them into a separate clean bowl, then add the blackberries, 2 tablespoons of sugar, 2 teaspoons of lemon juice and mix.

2. Scoop the fruit mixture into the oven dish and spread it out.

3. Put flour, a pinch of salt, sugar, the butter, 1 tablespoon cold water in a clean bowl and mix together with your fingertips until you have a crumbly mixture.

4. Preheat the Air fryer to 390°F.

5. Evenly distribute the flour mixture over the fruit.

6. Put the oven dish into the basket and slide the basket into the Air Fryer.

7. Set the fryer to cook for 20 minutes.

Mozzarella Sticks

COOKING ITEMS

Mozzarella cheese,

1 piece of Egg

Nonfat milk

White Flour (0.25 cup)

A cup of plain breadcrumbs

INSTRUCTIONS

1) Cut cheese into 3, each slice, should be 1/2 an inch stick.
2) Place breadcrumbs in a bowl, add the egg and milk to the bowl and stir
3) Dip cheese sticks into the mixture.
4) Lay breaded sticks on a cookie sheet.
5) And place into a freezer until solid.
6) Preheat the fryer
7) Place small batches of breaded sticks Basket and place into the fryer (note, try not to overlap)
8) Press the M Button and scroll to the French Fries Icon.
9) Press the Power Button & set the fryer to cook at 400 degrees for 5-10 minute, periodically check to stay acquainted with cooking texture.

AIR FRYER PORK, BEEF & LAMB RECIPES

Breaded Pork Chops

COOKING ITEMS:

Olive oil spray

6 centers cut boneless pork chops (thinly sliced)

Fat trimmed (5 ounces each)

½and ¾ teaspoon of Kosher Salt

1 egg

Half a cup of panko crumbs

Crushed cornflakes crumbs (1/3 cup)

Grated parmesan cheese (2 tablespoons)

Sweet paprika (1 ¼ teaspoons)

Garlic powder (½ teaspoon)

Onion powder (use ½ a teaspoon)

Chili powder (use ¼ a teaspoon)

Black pepper (use 1/8 a teaspoon)

INSTRUCTIONS:

1) Preheat the air fryer to 400F and lightly spray the basket with the olive oil.

2) Season pork chops with 1/2 teaspoons of kosher salt.

3) Combine panko, cornflake crumbs, parmesan cheese, and 3/4 teaspoon of kosher salt, paprika, garlic powder, onion powder, chili powder and black pepper in a bowl.

4) Break the egg into another bowl and beat till smooth. Dip the pork into the egg, and then dip into the crumb mixture as well.

5) Place chops into the basket and spritz the top with oil.

6) Put the basket into the fryer and cook for 12 minutes, turn halfway while it cooks and, set aside and repeat with the remaining.

Air Fryer Chinese Salt & Pepper Pork Chops

COOKING ITEMS

Pork Chops

1 piece of egg (you need the egg white, not the yolk)

Sea salt (use1/2 teaspoon)

Ground black pepper (use 1/4 teaspoon)

Potato starch or cornstarch (3/4 cup)

1 oil mister

STIR FRY

2 jalapeño pepper (stems must be removed, sliced)

2 scallions green onions (to be trimmed and sliced)

Canola oil or peanut (use 2 tablespoons)

1 teaspoon of sea salt

Ground black pepper (1/4 teaspoon)

Cast iron chicken fryer

INSTRUCTIONS

1) Spray air fryer basket with oil Coat

2) In a separate clean bowl, whisk egg white, salt, and pepper until smooth.

3) Slice pork chops into cutlet pieces, leaving a little on the bone and pat dry

4) Pour egg white mixture into pork chops and mix well to coat.

5) Set aside in a cool place and let it marinate for 20 minutes or more.

6) After 20 minutes, add pork chops to potato starch and dredge the pork chops through the starch.

7) Place pork in prepared Air Fryer Basket and lightly spray pork with Oil.

8) Set the fryer to Cook for 10-12 minutes 200 degrees.

9) Periodically shake the pork chops to ensure even cooking until the pork becomes brown

STIR FRY

10) Slice Jalapeños pepper and remove seeds.

11) Chop scallions, place in a bowl and set aside.

12) Heat up the skillet and add oil, Jalapeño peppers, Scallions, salt, pepper, and stir-fry for about a minute.

13) Add air fried pork pieces to the skillet and toss in the Jalapeño, Scallions, and stir-fry making sure they become coated with the hot oil and vegetables.

Beef Empanadas

COOKING ITEMS

Ground beef (1 pound)

Packaged empanada shells

Olive oil (2-3 tablespoons)

Green peppers (use 1 piece, seeded and diced into chunks)

Onion, peeled and minced

Clove garlic, peeled and minced

Half teaspoon of cumin

A quarter cup of tomato salsa

Sea salt

Pepper

Egg yolk

INSTRUCTIONS

1) Preheat sauté pan, add oil, ground beef and cook until all the meat is browned. Discard any excess fat, and then add garlic and onions and cover to cook for 4 minutes.

2) Add other cooking items except for the egg, milk and empanada shells.

3) Stir and let it cook for 10 minutes on low heat.

4) In a separate clean bowl mix egg and milk together.

5) Place an empanada shell on a clean counter. Add some of the cooked meat on one half of the rolled dough.

6) Brush the edges with egg wash and fold over. Seal open edges by merging with a fork. Brush with egg wash and place into the Fry Basket.

6) Repeat the process for the rest of the items

7) Place the Basket into the air fryer, Press the M Button, scroll to the Roast Icon, Press the Power Button and set the fryer to cook at 350 degrees for 10 minutes.

Beef Roll Up

COOKING ITEMS

Beef flank steak (2 pounds)

Pesto (3 tablespoons)

Provolone cheese (6 slices)

3 ounce of roasted red bell peppers,

Fresh baby spinach, (1/4 cup)

Sea Salt (1 teaspoon)

Black pepper (1 teaspoon)

INSTRUCTIONS

1) Open up the beef flank steak and spread the pesto evenly on the meat.

2) Layer the cheese, roasted red peppers & spinach 3/4 of the way down the meat.

3) Roll up the meat and secure with toothpicks, then season with sea salt and pepper.

4) Place the roll-ups in the Fry Basket and place the basket into the Air Fryer

5) If using the power XL air fryer, Press the M Button, scroll to the Steak Icon.

6) Press the Power Button & set the fryer to cools for 14 minutes at 400 degrees.

7) Rotate the meat after seven minutes

8) When cooked, set aside for ten minutes

9) Serving and enjoy

Air Fryer Pork Taquitos Recipe

COOKING ITEMS

Shredded pork tenderloin or shredded chicken (3 ounces)

Fat-free shredded mozzarella (2 ½ cups)

Flour tortillas (10 small)

1 lime (juiced)

Cooking spray

Salsa

Sour cream

INSTRUCTIONS

1) Place shredded chicken or pork in a bowl sprinkle some lime juice over pork and gently mix around.

2) Microwave 5 tortillas, set aside and damp paper towel over it for 10 seconds.

3) Add 3 oz. Of the meat and 1/4 cup of cheese to a tortilla and roll up the tortilla.

4) Line tortillas on a greased foil, spray cooking spray over the tortilla and place into the basket

5) Preheat air fryer.

6) Place basket into air fryer

7) Set the fryer to cook for 10 minutes at 400 degrees Celsius.

8) When cooked, turn off the fryer, dish and serve.

Lamb Chops with Garlic Sauce

COOKING ITEM

1 garlic bulb

Olive oil (3 tablespoons)

1 tablespoon of finely chopped fresh oregano

Sea salt

Freshly ground black pepper (1/2 teaspoon)

8 pieces of lamb chops

INSTRUCTIONS

1) Coat the garlic bulb with olive oil and put it in the basket.

2) Preheat the fryer

3) Slide the basket into the air fryer and set the fryer to cook for 12 minutes. After that, remove and set aside.

4) In a clean bowl, mix the fresh oregano with some sea salt, pepper, and olive oil.

5) Thinly coat the lamb chops with half a tablespoon of olive oil and set aside for 5 minutes.

6) Pre-heat the air fryer to 200°C.

7) Place four pieces of lamb chops into the basket, slide the basket into the air fryer, and set the timer to cook for 5 minutes, for the lambs to roast.

8) Place the remaining into fryer and roast for another 5 minutes.

9) Squeeze the garlic cloves between thumb and index finger over the herb oil. Add some salt and pepper, and stir the mixture well.

10) Serve the lamb chops with garlic sauce.

11) Garnish with couscous and braised zucchini.

Easy recipe for air fryer lamb chop

COOKING ITEMS:

4 pieces of Lamb Chops

Olive Oil (1 1/2 tablespoons)

1/2 tablespoons of finely chopped Fresh Oregano

A clove of Garlic

Salt

Ground Black Pepper

INSTRUCTIONS:

1) Preheat the air fryer to 200°C, then coat the clove of garlic with olive oil and put it in a fryer basket, place basket into the air fryer, then roast the garlic for 12 minutes and set aside.

2) In a separate bowl, mix the herbs with some salt, pepper and olive oil. Thinly coat the 4 lamb chops with half of the herb oil and leave them for 3 minutes.

3) Preheat the air fryer to 200°C, and Place four lamb chops into the basket.

4) Roast the lamb chops for 5 minutes till nicely brown and set aside.

5) Squeeze the garlic cloves between thumb and index finger over the herb oil. Add some salt and pepper, and stir the mixture well.

6) Garnish the lamb chops with garlic sauce.

7) Serve and Enjoy.

Air Fried Rack of Lamb

COOKING ITEMS

Frenched Rack of Lamb (1.5 pounds)

Mustard

Panko breadcrumbs

Rosemary

Oregano

Salt

Pepper

Extra Virgin Olive Oil

INSTRUCTIONS

1) Put all items except mustard and lamb into a food processor.

2) Blend until desired consistency is gotten.

3) Spray your air fryer basket with oil and then place lamb inside.

4) Put basket into air fryer and set fry to cook at 380 degrees for 17-18

5) Periodically brush the meat with mustard and rub the seasonings mixture on it.

Easy Greek Lamb, Spinach Meatballs with Tzatziki

COOKING ITEMS

Meatballs

1 lb. Of ground lamb

Packed chopped spinach (2 cups)

2 cloves of garlic (to be minced)

Minced onion (1 cup)

Chopped pine nuts (1/3 cup)

1 piece of egg

Olive oil (1 tablespoon)

Finely minced fresh oregano (1 tablespoon)

Finely crumbled feta (1/2 cup)

Salt (1/2 teaspoon)

TZATZIKI

1 cup full-fat plain Greek yogurt

Diced cucumber (1/3 cup)

Chopped fresh dill (2 tablespoons)

Chopped fresh mint (2 tablespoons)

Lemon juice (2 teaspoons)

Olive oil (1 teaspoon)

1-2 cloves garlic

Salt (1/4 teaspoon)

INSTRUCTIONS

1. Using a sauté pan, pour in oil and heat it up until shimmering.

2. Add minced onions and cook on medium-low heat until thoroughly.

3. Add minced garlic and cook for another 2-3 minutes.

4. Add chopped spinach and cook for another 4-5 minutes, until the spinach is wilted and some of the liquid cooks off and then set aside.

5. Put spinach mixture with the lamb, feta, pine nuts, oregano, and salt in a large bowl, then mix thoroughly mix all items.

6. Preheat the Air Fryer.

7. Place the meatballs into the fryer basket and cook for 11 minutes at 200 degree Celsius until brown.

8. Combine all the cooking items for the tzatziki in a small bowl and mix thoroughly.

9. Serve with meatballs

Air Fryer Chinese Sweet 'N Sour Pork

COOKING ITEMS

Pork meats (use 2 pounds and cut into chunks)

Eggs (2 pieces)

Pure Sesame Oil (1 teaspoon)

Cornstarch (1 cup)

Sea Salt (half teaspoon)

Freshly Ground Black Pepper (1/4 teaspoon)

Chinese Five Spice (1/16 teaspoon)

Canola Oil (3 Tablespoons)

OTHER

Oil Mister

1 prepared Simple Sweet 'N Sour Sauce Recipe

INSTRUCTIONS

1. Combine the potato starch, salt, pepper and Chinese Five Spice into a clean bowl, and set aside.

2. Beat the eggs in a separate clean bowl and add Sesame Oil.

3. Dredge the pork pieces into the Potato Starch and shake off any excess, then dip each piece into the egg mixture, shake off excess and then back into the Potato Starch mixture.

4. Coat Air Fryer Basket with oil, then place pork pieces into the basket and spray oil on the pork and put the basket into the fryer.

5. Cook at 340 degrees for approximately 8-12 minutes; periodically shake the basket to ensure that meal is evenly cooked.

6. Dish with any kind of sauce of your choice

7. Serve and enjoy.

CHICKEN/POULTRY RECIPES

Jerk Chicken Wings

COOKING ITEMS:
Chicken wings (use 3 pounds)
Olive oil (use 2 tablespoons)
Soy sauce (use 2 tablespoons)
6 cloves of garlic (minced)
1 habanero pepper, seeds and ribs removed, finely chopped
Allspice (use 1 tablespoon)
Cinnamon (use 1 teaspoon)
Cayenne pepper (use 1 teaspoon)
White pepper (use 1 teaspoon)
Salt (1 teaspoon)
Brown sugar (use 2 tablespoons)
Finely chopped fresh thyme (use 1 tablespoon)
Grated fresh ginger (use 1 tablespoon)
4 finely chopped scallions
Lime juice (use 5 tablespoons)
Red wine vinegar (use ½ a cup)

INSTRUCTIONS:
1) Combine all the cooking items into a large clean bowl, garnish with seasoning
2) Place in a cool place for 20 minutes to marinade.
3) Transfer to a 1-gallon re-sealable bag and refrigerate for 2 hours up to 24 hours.
4) Preheat the air fryer to 390°f.
5) Remove the bag from the fridge, remove the wings, and pat the wings completely dry with a paper towel.
6) Place the wings into the cooking basket, place basket into the fryer and cook for 16-18 minutes, shaking halfway through.

7) Dish with blue cheese or ranch dressing.

8) Serve and enjoy.

Hot Wings

COOKING ITEMS

12 chicken wings

Brunettes raw

Buffalo sauce (1 cup)

INSTRUCTIONS

1. Preheat the fryer
2. Place the wings into the Fry Basket and put the basket into the fryer.
3. If using the Power Air Fryer XL, Press the M Button and scroll to the French Fries Icon and press the Power Button, then adjust the fryer to cook for 25 minutes at 400 degrees Celsius.
4. Periodically check the wings and shake to enable even frying
5. When done remove the basket, toss the wings in sauce, and mix
6. Return the wings to the fryer, Press the M Button. Scroll to the French Fries Icon and cook for another 8 more minutes at 400 degrees.
7. Toss halfway through to ensure even cooking
8. Serve and enjoy

Chicken Tenders

COOKING ITEMS

Chicken tender (6 pieces)

3 pieces of large eggs

A half cup of white Flour

White

1 cup of panko

1 teaspoon of sea salt

Half teaspoon of black pepper

1 teaspoon olive oil

A half cup of milk

INSTRUCTIONS

1) Put panko breadcrumbs in a separate bowl add olive oil, and mix.

2) Pour egg into a bowl and whisk

3) Put the white flour and milk in a separate clean bowl and mix.

4) Dip chicken tenders into the flour, then into the panko mixture, and finally into the egg mixture.

5) Place breaded tenders into the Fry Basket. Repeat until done.

6) Place the Fry Basket into Air Fryer. If using the power XL fryer, Press the M button and scroll to the French Fries Icon.

7) Set fryer to cook for 14 minutes at 400 degrees Celsius.

8) Periodically check and flip for even cooking.

9) Serve and Enjoy with your favorite dipping sauce.

Air Fryer Chicken Sandwich

COOKING ITEMS

2 boneless chicken Breasts

Dill Pickle Juice (use 2 cups)

2 pieces of Eggs

Milk (use ½ a cup)

All-Purpose Flour (use 1 cup)

Powdered Sugar (use 2 tablespoons)

Paprika (use 1 teaspoon)

Sea Salt (use 1 teaspoon)

Ground Black Pepper (½ teaspoon)

Garlic Powder (½ teaspoon)

Ground Celery Seed ground (use ¼ a teaspoon)

Extra Virgin Olive Oil (use 1 Tablespoon)

1 Oil Mister

4 Hamburger Buns, buttered and toasted

Pickle Chips

SPICY OPTION

1/4 teaspoon Cayenne Pepper

INSTRUCTIONS

1) Place chicken in a Ziploc Bag and pound, so that the whole piece has the same thickness, of about ½ inch thick and slice each chicken breast into two or three pieces

2) Place chicken back into Ziploc baggie, pour in pickle juice and place into the refrigerator for at least 30 minutes to marinate

3) Break egg into a clean bowl; add some milk and whisk until smooth.

4) In another bowl, combine 1 cup of flour and the rest of the spices and mix well.

5) Coat the chicken with the egg mixture and then into flour mixture, and make sure pieces are lightly and completely coated.

6) Preheat air fryer, and spray the bottom of your Air Fryer basket with Oil.

7) Place the basket of chicken into air fryer and spray the chicken with a little Oil.

8) Set the fryer to Cook at 340 degrees for 10-15 minutes and periodically shake the chicken to ensure even cooking

9) Serve and garnish with buttered and toasted buns and a dollop of mayonnaise

Roast Turkey Breast

COOKING ITEMS

Turkey breast (use 8 pounds)

Sea Salt (use 2 tablespoons)

Black pepper (use 1 tablespoon)

Olive oil (2 tablespoons)

INSTRUCTIONS

1) Put the turkey in a separate bowl, season the turkey and rub with olive oil.

2) Preheat the air fryer.

3) Place the turkey breast side down in the Fry Basket.

4) Using the chicken icon, adjust cooking time to 40 minutes and set to cook at 200 degrees Celsius

5) After 20 minutes turn the breasts over and let the remaining 20 minutes timer to exhaust.

6) Ensure meat is properly cooked to your taste if not, you can let it cook for another 5 to 10 minutes in the fryer

7) Set aside for 20 minutes

8) Serving and enjoy.

Chicken Pot Pie

COOKING ITEMS

6 Chicken tenders

1½ cup cream of condensed celery soup,

2 potatoes, peeled and diced

Quarter cup heavy Cream

1 dried bay leaf

1 sprig of thyme

1 piece of egg

Milk (1 tablespoon)

obuttermilk biscuit dough for 5 biscuits

INSTRUCTIONS

1) Put all items except the biscuits, egg yolk, and milk into a clean pot, place on the gas stove and bring to a boil

2) Pour the items into a baking pan and cover with foil, then place the pan into the Fryer Basket and place the basket into the air fryer

3) Using the Bake Icon, adjust the fryer to cook for 15 minutes at 320 degrees.

4) Mix the egg yolk and milk together in a separate clean bowl to make an egg wash.

5) When the timer runs out, open the fryer and add the biscuits to the Baking Pan. Brush the biscuits with egg wash and Place the baking pan back into the Fry Basket.

6) Set the fryer to cook for another 10 minutes at 300 degrees.

7) Turn off the fryer, bring out the pan and dish

8) Serve and enjoy

Air Fried Crumbed Chicken Tenderloins

COOKING ITEMS

1 piece of egg

Dry bread crumbs (use ½ a cup)

Vegetable oil (use 2 tablespoons)

Chicken tenderloins (8 pieces)

INSTRUCTIONS

1) Whisk the egg into a small clean bowl.

2) Pour bread crumbs into another clean bowl, put in some oil and mix until crumbly.

3) Dip each chicken piece of tenderloin into the bowl of egg, then into the crumb mixture.

4) First Preheat an air fryer to 350 degrees F

5) Place chicken in the air fryer basket and place basket into the fryer

6) Cook for 12 minutes.

7) Serve and enjoy

Air Fryer Chicken Nuggets

COOKING ITEMS:

2 large boneless chicken breasts, (slice into even 1-inch bite-sized pieces)

Olive oil (2 teaspoons)

Whole wheat Italian breadcrumbs (6 tablespoons)

Panko (2 tablespoons)

Grated parmesan cheese (2 tablespoons)

Olive oil spray

Black pepper

Kosher salt (1/2 teaspoon)

INSTRUCTIONS:

1) Put breadcrumb, olive oil, 2 tablespoons of panko and parmesan cheese in another.

2) Put chicken in bowl and season with salt, olive oil, and pepper, and mix well with ingredients to coat with chicken

3) Coat chicken in breadcrumbs, and place into the basket.

4) Preheat air fryer to cook to 400°F for 8 minutes.

5) Place basket into the fryer and air fry for 10 minutes

6) Periodically check to enable even cooking.

7) Cook for another 5 if desired tenderness is not reached.

8) Dish and serve

Air Fryer Chicken Kiev Supper

COOKING ITEMS

Chicken Breast

Soft Cheese garlic (100 grams)

Garlic Puree (1/4 teaspoon)

Parsley (1 Teaspoon)

1 piece of egg

Breadcrumbs

Herb flavor

Salt

Pepper

INSTRUCTIONS

1. Put ½ teaspoon of parsley into a bowl; add the garlic and the soft cheese.

2. Put bread crumbs herb flavor, ½ teaspoon of parsley salt and pepper and mix

3. Flatten chicken breast with rolling pin and slice into 2 equal parts.

4. Place the mixture in between the sliced breasts the clap the two chicken breasts together.

5. Break the egg into a separate bowl.

6. Dip the chicken into the bowl of egg and into the bowl of breadcrumbs

7. Preheat the fryer

8. Cook on a 180c heat in the Air Fryer for 25 minutes

9. Periodically check and turn to ensure even cooking.

10. Dish and Serve.

Air Fried KFC Popcorn Chicken

COOKING ITEMS

1 Chicken Breast

KFC Spice Blend (2 ml)

Bread Crumbs (60 ml)

1 piece of egg

White Flour (50 gram)

Salt

Pepper

INSTRUCTIONS

1) Put chicken into a food processor, blend and set aside.

2) Pour white flour into a clean bowl

3) Break egg into the second bowl and whisk.

4) Pour KFC spice blend, salt and pepper and breadcrumbs into the third bowl.

5) Rub flour on your palm and make your minced chicken into balls and roll in the bowl of flour, in a bowl of egg and finally in the spiced breadcrumbs.

6) Preheat air fryer and place the chicken balls into the fryer basket.

7) Set fryer to cook at 180c for 12-15 minutes

8) Dish and serve

Easy Airfryer KFC Chicken Strips

COOKING ITEMS

1 boneless Chicken Breast

Desiccated Coconut (15 ml)

Plain Oats (15 ml)

KFC Spice Blend (5 ml)

Bread Crumbs (75 ml)

White Plain Flour (50g)

1 piece of egg

Salt

Pepper

INSTRUCTIONS

1) Chop chicken breast into strips and put into a clean bowl.

2) Put a mixture of coconut, oats, KFC spice blend, bread crumbs, salt and pepper into a bowl.

3) Break eggs into a clean bowl.

4) Put flour into another

5) Dip chicken strips into the plain flour, then in the egg and finally in the bowl spice mixture.

6) Pre-heat the fryer

7) Place in the Air fryer at 180c and cook for 12 minutes

8) When cooked, dish and Serve.

Zinger Chicken Burger

COOKING ITEMS

6 pieces of Chicken Breasts

1 piece of egg

Plain Flour (50 gram)

KFC Spice Blend (10 ml)

Bread Crumbs (100 ml)

Worcester sauce (1 teaspoon)

Mustard Powder (1 teaspoon)

Paprika (1 teaspoon)

Salt

Pepper

INSTRUCTIONS

1) Put chicken, Worcester sauce, mustard, paprika and salt and pepper into food processor and blend

2) Rub a little powder on your palm, make the chicken into burger shapes and set aside.

3) Break the eggs into a bowl.

4) Pour flour into another bowl.

5) Pour the KFC spice blend and bread crumbs into another.

6) Dip the burgers in the flour, the egg and then the breadcrumbs.

7) Preheat the air fryer and place burger in the fryer basket

8) Place basket in the Air fryer set to cook at 180c for 15 minutes

9) When the timer beeps, dish and serve

FISH/SEAFOOD

Air Fryer 3 Ingredient Fried Catfish

COOKING ITEMS

4 pieces of catfish

Seasoned fish fry (1/4 cup)

Olive oil (1 teaspoon)

Chopped parsley (1 teaspoon)

INSTRUCTIONS

1) Rinse the 4 catfishes and slice into fillets.

2) Pour the fish fillets into a large Ziploc bag.

3) Put the catfish into the bag, and seal the bag

4) Shake to ensure the entire filet is coated with seasoning

5) Spray olive oil on the top of each filet.

6) Preheat Air Fryer to 400 degrees.

7) Place the fillet in the Air Fryer basket

8) Set fryer to cook for 20 minutes.

9) Check after 10 minutes and flip for even frying

10) Dish, garnish with parsley and serve.

Air-fryer Fish & Chips

COOKING ITEMS:

1 pack fries (for four)

2 fish fillets

1 piece of egg

3-4 slices wheat bread (died and made into breadcrumbs)

Tortilla chips (25g bag)

1 lemon (juiced)

Parsley (1 tablespoon)

Salt

Pepper

INSTRUCTIONS

1) Prepare the fries.

2) Divide the 2 fish fillets into four equal pieces and season with lemon juice and then put to one side.

3) Break egg into a clean bowl

4) Put breadcrumbs, lemon rind, parsley, tortillas and salt and pepper into food processor. Pour into a bowl.

5) Dip fish in the bowl of beaten egg and then dip into the bowl of breadcrumbs mixture.

6) Cook for 15 minutes on 180°C until nice and crispy

7) Dish and serve

Air Fried Crumbed Fish

COOKING ITEMS

Vegetable oil (4 tablespoons)

Breadcrumbs (100g)

1 piece of egg

4 fish fillets

1 lemon

INSTRUCTIONS

1) Put oil and breadcrumbs together in a clean bowl and stir until the mixture becomes loose and crumbly.

2) Pre-heat your air fryer to 180 degrees C.

3) Dip the fish fillets into the egg then shake off any residual, then into the crumb mix making sure it is evenly and fully covered.

4) Gently place the fryer basket and set the air fryer to cook for 15 minutes.

5) Dish immediately and serve with lemon.

Air-fryer Fried Cod Fish

COOKING ITEMS

Codfish of 200 grams

Sesame oil

1 cup of water

Light soy sauce (5 tablespoons)

Dark soy sauce (1 teaspoon)

Rock sugar (5 cubes)

Olive oil (3 tablespoons)

5 slices of ginger

Spring onions (shredded)

Coriander

Salt

Sugar

INSTRUCTIONS:

1) Wash the fish codfish and place in a clean dry bowl, then season with salt sugar and a dash of sesame oil

2) Preheat your air-fryer for 3 minutes at 180°C.

3) Place fish in fryer basket and Air-fry codfish for 12 minutes.

4) Pour light soy sauce, dark soy sauce, rock sugar, hot water into a bowl and stir till the sugar melts.

5) Put oil into a sauté pan to heat up; add ginger and white part of spring onion. And fry till ginger turns brown.

6) Remove ginger and spring onion from the oil.

7) Place cod fish into a dish and top with garnish, then pour the boiling oil over the fish. Spoon seasoning sauce over the fish.

8) Serve immediately and enjoy.

Cod Fish Nuggets

COOKING ITEMS

1 pound cod

FOR THE BREADING:

Olive oil (2 tablespoons)

All-purpose flour (1 cup)

2 pieces of eggs,

¾ cup panko breadcrumbs

Salt

INSTRUCTIONS:

1) Cut the cod into strips approximately

2) Blend the panko breadcrumbs, olive oil and salt to a fine crumb in a food processor.

3) Put panko mixture into a separate bowl,

4) Break eggs in a separate bowl and whisk

5) Pour flour into another bowl

6) Separate dip each piece of cod into the flour, then the eggs and then the breadcrumbs.

7) Dip the fish firmly into breadcrumbs.

8) Shake off any excess breadcrumbs.

9) Preheat the Air fryer to 180°c.

10) Add the cod nuggets to the fryer basket, and cook for 8-10 minutes.

Air-Fried Fish & Chips with Tangy Herb Sauce

COOKING ITEMS

FRIES:

2 Russet potatoes (sliced into sticks)

2 teaspoons canola oil

Kosher salt

FISH:

Flour (1/4 cup)

1 piece of egg

1 teaspoon of Dijon mustard

Seasoned panko bread crumbs (3/4 cup)

Canola oil (2½ Teaspoons)

4 cod fish fillets (about 6 ounces)

SAUCE:

Light mayonnaise (1/4 cup)

Light plain yogurt (2 tablespoons)

Chopped dill pickle (2 tablespoons)

Chopped red onion (2 tablespoons)

Chopped dill (1 tablespoon)

Chopped tarragon (1 tablespoon)

Capers (2 teaspoons)

INSTRUCTIONS

FRIES:

1) Soak potato sticks in water for 30 minutes and drain.

2) Preheat air fryer at 200 degrees Celsius for 3 minutes.

3) Put oil in the bowl of potato and mix until well coated.

4) Put into fryer basket, place basket into the fryer and set to cook for 20 to 25 minutes,

5) Periodically shake to enable even frying.

FISH:

1) Set fryer at 370 degrees.

2) Spread flour on waxed paper.

3) Break egg into a bowl and add mustard.

4) Pour breadcrumbs into a bowl, add oil and mix well.

5) Coat fish in flour, then egg mixture, then crumbs and place in fryer basket.

6) Set fryer to cook for 10 minutes

SAUCE:

1) Combine all sauce cooking items in a small bowl and mix well.

2) Serve with fish and fries.

Air-fryer Salmon Fishcakes Crumb

COOKING ITEMS:

Salmon (250 grams)

400g of mashed potato

Capers (1 handful)

Chopped parsley

Zest of 1 lemon

Plain flour (2 ounces)

Spray oil

Salt

Pepper

INSTRUCTIONS:

1) Flake the salmon; add mashed potato, capers, dill, zest and Season.

2) Shape into small cakes and dust with flour. Chill in the fridge for 1 hour to firm up.

3) Heat the air-fryer to 180°C.

4) Place the fishcakes in the fryer basket,

5) Spray with oil and cook for 7 minutes.

Grilled fish fillet with pesto sauce

COOKING ITEMS

Whitefish fillets (3 pieces of 200 grams each)

Olive oil (1 tablespoon)

1 bunch fresh basil (15 g)

2 garlic cloves

Pinenuts (2 tablespoons)

Grated parmesan cheese (1 tablespoon)

1 cup extra virgin olive oil

Pepper

Salt

INSTRUCTIONS

1) Put fillet into a clean bowl, add oil and garnish with pepper and salt.

2) Preheat the Air fryer to 180°c.

3) Place fish fillets in the fryer basket, slide the basket into the Air fryer and set the timer for 8 to 10 minutes.

4) Put basil leaves, garlic, salt, pine nuts, parmesan cheese and olive oil and place in food processor.

5) Blend the mixture until smooth

6) Place the fish fillets on a serving plate and serve them drizzled with the pesto sauce.

Avocado Fries

COOKING ITEMS

Panko breadcrumbs (1/2 cup)

Salt

Haas avocado (1 piece, peeled, pitted, and sliced)

Aquafaba from 115-ounce garbanzo beans

INSTRUCTION

1) Put panko and salt into a clean bowl.

2) Pour the aquafaba into another bowl.

3) Dip the avocado slices in the aquafaba and then in the panko.

4) Arrange the avocado slices into a single layer in your air fryer basket.

5) Place the basket into the fryer

6) Air fry for 10 minutes at 390F,

7) Periodically check and shake well to ensure even frying.

8) Dish immediately with any dipping sauce or burrito

Guilt-Free Air fryer Vegetable Fries

COOKING ITEMS

Sweet Potato (150 grams)

Courgette (150 grams)

Carrots (150 grams)

Olive Oil (2 Tablespoons)

Thyme (1 Teaspoon)

Pinch Mixed Spice

Pinch Basil

Salt

Pepper

INSTRUCTIONS

1) Peel sweet potatoes and place into a clean bowl of water.

2) Peel carrots and set aside

3) Chop up the sweet potato, the carrots, and the courgettes into chunky chips shape.

4) Preheat air fryer

5) Pour into fryer basket, add olive oil and cook for 18 minutes at 180c at 12 minutes

6) Periodically shake to ensure even cooking.

7) Once cooked place, pour into round bowl and add the seasoning.

8) Shake well, dish and serve.

Air Fryer Ranch Kale Chips

COOKING ITEMS

Olive oil (2 tablespoons)

Loosely packed kale stemmed (4 cups)

Vegan ranch seasoning (2 teaspoons)

Nutritional yeast flakes (1 tablespoon)

Salt

INSTRUCTION

1) Stem kale on gas and set aside

2) Pour kale pieces, Ranch Seasoning, oil, and nutritional yeast in a clean bowl, and shake well to coat

3) Put the coated kale into the basket of your air fryer.

4) Cook on 180 degree Celsius for 5-6 minutes,

5) Periodically shake, to ensure even cooking.

6) Dish and serve immediately.

Curried Sweet Potato Oven Fries with Creamy Cumin Ketchup

COOKING ITEMS

FOR THE SWEET POTATO FRIES
2 pieces of sweet potatoes

Olive oil (use 2-3 tablespoons)

Curry powder (use 1/2 teaspoon)

Coriander (use 1/4 teaspoon)

Sea salt (use 1/4 teaspoon)

FOR THE CREAMY CUMIN KETCHUP

Ketchup (1/2 a cup)

Vegan mayo (use 2 tablespoons)

 Ground cumin (1/2 tablespoon)

Ground ginger (use 1/8 teaspoon)

Cinnamon (a pinch)

INSTRUCTION

Separately make the sweet potato fries

1) Cut your sweet potatoes into tiny slices

2) Arrange the sweet potato slices on a cookie sheet, and drizzle 2 tablespoons of the olive oil, and sprinkle curry powder, coriander, and sea salt.

3) Toss well to ensure even coating.

4) Preheat air fryer

5) Transfer the sweet potato fries to your air fryer basket.

6) Cook at 370F for 20 minutes

7) Periodically check and shake after 10 minutes.

Make the Creamy Cumin Ketchup

8) Put the ketchup items together in a small bowl and whisk

Air Fryer Tofu Scramble

COOKING ITEMS

A block of tofu chopped (chopped)

Soy sauce (use 2 tablespoons)

Olive oil (use 1 tablespoon)

Turmeric (use 1 teaspoon)

 Garlic powder (use ½ a teaspoon)

Onion powder (use ½ a teaspoon)

Chopped onion (use ½ cup)

2-3 pieces of potatoes (sliced)

Olive oil (1 tablespoon)

Broccoli florets (4 cups)

INSTRUCTION

1) Toss the tofu, soy sauce, olive oil, turmeric, garlic powder, onion powder, and onion. Then Set aside in a cool place to marinate.

2) Preheat air fryer

3) Toss oil into potatoes, pour into fryer basket, air fry at 400F for 15 minutes,

4) Periodically check and shake to ensure even frying.

5) After 15 minutes, add tofu to the potatoes and shake

6) Set the fryer to cook at 370 for 15 more minutes.

7) While the tofu is cooking, toss the broccoli in the reserved marinade. If there isn't enough to get it all over the broccoli, add a little bit of extra soy sauce.

8) Add broccoli only when it is 2-3 minutes to the stoppage time

Healthy Mediterranean Vegetables

COOKING ITEMS

Cherry Tomatoes (50 grams)

Courgette (1 large piece)

Green Pepper (1 piece)

1 A large piece of Parsnip

1 piece of Carrot

Mixed Herbs (use 1 teaspoon)

Honey (use 2 tablespoons)

Mustard (use 1 teaspoon)

Garlic Puree (use 2 teaspoons)

Olive Oil (use 6 tablespoons)

Salt

Pepper

INSTRUCTIONS

1) Slice up the courgette, green pepper, Peel and dice the parsnip, whole tomatoes cherry and carrot in a clean bow an mix

2) Preheat air fryer

3) Drizzle with three tablespoons of olive oil and pour vegetable mixture into baking dish, place baking dish into fryer set fryer to cook at 180c for 15 minutes

4) In the meantime mix up the rest of your cooking items into a bowl

5) When the timer beeps, pull out the baking dish, pour in the mixture and shake well so that all the vegetables are covered in the marinade.

6) Sprinkle with a little more salt and pepper and cook for another 5 minutes at 200c.

7) Dish and Serve.

Cauliflower Veggie Burger Recipe

COOKING ITEMS

Cauliflower (1 kilo)

Coconut Oil (3 teaspoons)

Garlic Puree (2 teaspoons)

Bread Crumbs (1 Cup)

Desiccated Coconut (use quarter)

Oats (use ½ a cup)

Plain Flour (3 tablespoons)

1 piece of Egg

Herby Bread Crumbs (use 2 cups)

Mustard Powder (1 teaspoon)

Thyme (2 teaspoons)

Parsley (use 2 teaspoons)

Chives (2 teaspoons)

Mixed Spice (1 teaspoon)

Salt

Pepper

INSTRUCTIONS

1) Mix two cups of plain bread crumbs with a teaspoon of salt, pepper, and parsley in a bowl, and set aside as herby breadcrumbs.

2) Chop cauliflower into florets, steam in a soup maker for 25 minutes

3) When steamed, drain the cauliflower and dice it, into small pieces.

4) Add to it salt, pepper, mustard and a teaspoon of garlic puree. Blend for a couple of minutes and then drain over the sink.

5) Place the cauliflower into a tea towel and drain out all the excess water

6) Place the drained cauliflower in a clean dry bowl; add salt, pepper, other seasonings, garlic puree, coconut oil, the desiccated coconut, oats and one cup of breadcrumbs.

7) Rub flour on your palm, so that it doesn't stick, mold the mixture and shape into burgers.

8) Break egg into a clean bowl and whisk, pour flour into another clean bowl, add bread crumbs in the third bowl.

9) Roll in the bugger mix in flour, egg and then the herby breadcrumbs

10) Place bugger into air fryer basket

11) Place the basket in the Air fryer and set to cook for 10 minutes on each side at 180c.

12) Serve garnished with salad and burger bun.

Cauliflower Cheese Tater Tots

COOKING ITEMS

Fresh Cauliflower (use 1 kilogram)

Cheddar Cheese (use 150 gram)

Bread Crumbs (use 100 ml)

Desiccated Coconut (use 15 ml)

Oats (use 15 ml)

1 piece of Egg

2 piece of onion (use thinly diced)

Garlic Puree (use 1 teaspoon)

Parsley (use 1 teaspoon)

Chives (use 1 teaspoon)

Oregano (use 1 teaspoon)

Salt

Pepper

INSTRUCTIONS

1) Chop your cauliflower and place into your soup maker and steam in a small quantity of water for 20 minutes

2) Mix the coconut, oats, and breadcrumbs in a bowl.

3) Break and beat the egg into a small clean bowl

4) When your cauliflower is cooked, drain it and place it into a clean bowl, add salt, pepper, garlic puree.

5) Place in food processor and blend till it resembles breadcrumbs. Place it into a clean tea towel and squeeze it for a few minutes until you have drained out the water.

6) Place the cauliflower back into the bowl, add onion, the rest of the herbs, the cheese and mix well.

7) Shape into tater tots and then roll in the bowl of egg and the bowl of breadcrumbs.

8) Place in the Air fryer basket and place basket into air fryer, set to cook for 6 minutes at 180c

9) When timer beeps, set to cook again for another 10 minutes at 200c

10) Dish and serve

Cheesy Potato Wedges

COOKING ITEMS

Potatoes (use 1 Pound)

Olive Oil (use 1 Teaspoon)

Salt (use 1 Teaspoon)

Ground Black Pepper (use 1 Teaspoon)

Garlic Powder (use 1/2 teaspoon)

CHEESE SAUCE

Raw cashews (use 1/2 cup)

Turmeric (use 1/2 teaspoon)

Paprika (use 1/2 teaspoon)

Nutritional yeast (use 2 tablespoons)

Lemon juice (use 1 teaspoon)

1/4 cup water

INSTRUCTIONS

1) Peel and slice potatoes into a bowl of water,

2) Drain water and add oil, salt pepper and garlic powder to the potatoes, then toss for potatoes to coat in spices.

3) Transfer the potatoes to the air fryer basket. Slide in the basket and set the fryer to cook for 16 minutes.

4) Periodically check and shake to ensure even cooking.

Cheese Sauce:

5) Put cashews, turmeric, paprika, nutritional yeast, and lemon juice into a food processor

6) Adding water as needed and blend into a cheese consistency.

7) Transfer the cooked potatoes to an air fryer pan.

8) Drizzle cheese sauce over the potatoes, place fryer into the pan and set to cook for 2-3 minutes at 200°c

9) Dish and serve

Kale and Potato Nuggets

COOKING ITEMS

Finely chopped potatoes

Olive oil or canola oil (use 1 teaspoon)

1 clove of garlic, (minced)

Loosely packed kale (4 cups, coarsely chopped)

Almond milk (1/8 cup)

Sea salt (1/4 teaspoon)

Ground black pepper (use 1/8 teaspoon)

Vegetable oil spray

INSTRUCTIONS

1) Cook the potatoes till it's soft.

2) Put oil in sauté pan and oil till shimmering, and then add onion and garlic till and sauté until brown.

3) Add the kale and sauté for 4-5 minutes then place into a bowl.

4) Place cooked potatoes into a bowl. Add mesh with a potato masher.

5) Pour kale into a bowl of mashed potatoes

6) Preheat the air fryer to 200°c for 5 minutes.

7) Spray the air fryer basket with vegetable oil.

8) Roll kale and potatoes into 1-inch nuggets

9) Place the nuggets in the air fryer

10) Slide basket into the fryer and let it cook for 12 to 15 minutes until golden brown

11) Periodically check to ensure even cooking.

12) Dish and serve

APPETIZERS AND SIDE DISHES

Fried Meatballs in Tomato Sauce

COOKING ITEMS:

Tomato sauce

A piece of onion

¾ pounds (12oz) ground beef

Chopped fresh parsley (1 tablespoon)

Chopped fresh thyme leaves (1/2 tablespoon)

A piece of egg

Breadcrumbs (3 tablespoons)

Pepper

Salt

10oz of your favorite tomato sauce

INSTRUCTIONS:

1) Chop onion and pour into a bowl, except tomato sauce, put the entire cooking item along with the onion and mix.

2) Preheat the Air fryer to 360 degree Celsius

3) Place the meatballs in the Air fryer basket, slide the basket into the Air fryer and set the fryer to cook for 8 minutes.

4) Transfer the meatballs to an oven dish, pour the tomato sauce over the meatballs and place the oven dish into the basket of the Air Fryer. Slide the basket into the Air Fryer.

5) Set the fryer to cook at 330°C and cook for five minutes

6) Dish and serve.

Air Fryer Cheddar Bacon Croquettes

COOKING ITEMS:

FOR THE FILLING:
Sharp cheddar cheese, block (use 1 pound)
Bacon, (use I pound, thinly sliced)

FOR THE BREADING:
Olive oil (4 tablespoons)
Cup all-purpose flour
Eggs (use 2 pieces)
Seasoned breadcrumbs (use 1 cup)

INSTRUCTIONS:
1) Slice cheddar cheese into 6 equally sized 1-inch portions
2) Rap two pieces of bacon around each piece of cheddar
3) Trim any excess fat.
4) Place the cheddar bacon bites in the freezer for 5 minutes
5) Pour oil and breadcrumbs into a bowl and mix until the mixture becomes crumbly.
6) Break egg into bowl and whisk, pour flour into another bowl and pour crumbs into the third bowl.
7) Put a little flower on your palms
8) Place each cheddar block into the flour, then the eggs and then the breadcrumbs. Press coating to croquettes
9) Preheat fryer to 200 degree Celsius
10) Place the croquettes in the cooking basket
11) Set fryer to cook for 8-10 minutes.
12) Periodically check to ensure that desired texture is achieved.
13) Dish and serve.

Air Fryer Roast Turkey Reuben

COOKING ITEMS
Boneless turkey breast (cut into 8 slices)

Rye Bread (4 slices)

Coleslaw (Use 4 tablespoons)

Salted butter (use 2 tablespoons)

8 slice of Swiss cheese

Russian dressing (use 2 tablespoons)

INSTRUCTIONS
1) Spread butter on 2 of the sliced bread.
2) Lay two slices of bread, on a cutting board, one on top of the other
3) Layer cheese, turkey, coleslaw and Russian dressing on top of each slice of bread.
4) Fold both halves together to make one sandwich.
5) Place into the Fry Basket
6) Slide in the fryer basket and adjust cooking time to 12 minutes at 310 degrees.
7) Check sandwich and turn over for even cooking.
8) Slice, dish, serve and enjoy

Air Fryer Peanut Butter Marshmallow Fluff

COOKING ITEMS

Filo pastry, defrosted (use 4 sheets)

Chunky peanut butter (use 4 tablespoons)

Marshmallow fluff (use 4 tablespoons)

Butter (use two ounces)

Sea salt

INSTRUCTIONS:

1) Preheat the Air fryer to 360°F.

2) Brush 1 sheet of filo pastry on a table and brush with butter,

3) Place the second sheet of filo on top of the first and brush with butter, do the same with third and fourth filo.

4) Cut the filo layers into 4 3-inches to 12-inches strips.

5) Place 1 tablespoon of peanut butter and 1 teaspoon of marshmallow fluff on the underside of a strip of filo.

6) Fold the tip of the sheet over the filling to form a triangle and fold repeatedly in a zigzag manner until the filling is fully wrapped.

7) Seal the ends together with a touch of butter.

8) Place into the cooking basket, slide basket into air fryer and cook for 5 minutes, until golden brown and puffy.

9) Lightly sprinkle sea salt when dishing

10) Serve and enjoy

Rosemary Russet Potato Chips

COOKING ITEMS:

Russet potatoes (use 4 pieces)

Olive oil (use 1 tablespoon)

2 teaspoons of chopped rosemary,

Sea salt

INSTRUCTIONS:

1) Peel the potatoes pour into a clean bowl of water and wash,

2) Slice into thin chips; pour directly into a bowl of water. Leave in water for 30 minutes.

3) Drain the water and pat completely dry

4) Put potatoes in mixing bowl, add olive oil and toss

5) Preheat the Air fryer to 330°F.

6) Place them in the cooking basket

7) Set fryer to cook for and 30 minutes at 330 200 degrees Celsius

8) Periodically check to ensure that it is golden brown.

9) When finished and still warm, toss in a large bowl with rosemary and salt.

10) Dish and serve

Air Fryer French Fries

COOKING ITEMS

Russet potatoes (2 pieces)

Olive oil (1 tablespoon)

Sea Salt (1 tablespoon)

Ground black pepper (Use ½ tablespoon)

INSTRUCTIONS

1) Peel potatoes and soak into a bowl of water until tender

2) Cut it into fries, and then toss with olive oil and salt and pepper.

3) Place the potatoes in the Fry Basket

4) Scroll to the French Fries Icon. And set to cook for 18 minutes at 400 degrees.

5) Periodically check and toss the fries to ensure even frying

6) Dish and serve

Air Fryer Stromboli

COOKING ITEMS

Pizza crust (use 12 ounces, place in the refrigerator)

3 cups of shredded cheddar cheese,

0.75 cup shredded Mozzarella cheese

0.333333 pound cooked ham, sliced

3 ounce of roasted red bell peppers

1 piece of egg

1 tablespoon of milk

INSTRUCTIONS

1. Roll the pizza dough out with a rolling pin until the dough is 1/4 inch thick.

2. Layer the ham, cheese, and peppers on one side of the dough and cover with the other side.

3. Break an egg, remove egg white and use the yolk, mix yolk with milk together in a bowl and brush the dough.

4. Place the Stromboli into the Fry Basket

6. Set fryer to cook for 15 minutes at 360 degrees, using chicken settings

7. Periodically turn to ensure that it is evenly cooked.

8. Dish and serve

DESSERTS & CAKES

Air Fryer Roast Chicken with Herbs

COOKING ITEMS

1 whole chicken of five pounds

Garlic powder (use 1 teaspoon)

Onion powder (use 1 teaspoon)

Sea salt (use I teaspoon)

Black pepper (use 1 teaspoon)

Thyme (use 1/2 teaspoon)

Olive oil (use 2 tablespoons)

INSTRUCTIONS

1. Place chicken into a clean bowl, add seasoning and olive oil and set aside for 45 minutes

2. Place the chicken in fryer basket.

3. Place basket into the fryer and set to cook for 40 minutes at 360 degrees

4. Check after 20 minutes and turn to the other side.

5. Cook for another 10 minutes if you want

6. Let rest for 20 minutes

7. Dish and serve

Air Fryer Donuts

COOKING ITEMS

Yeast (use ½ an ounce)

Low-fat milk (use ½ a cup)

Cinnamon (1/2 a teaspoon)

Unsalted butter (2 tablespoons)

Flour, white (use 2½ cup of flour)

Nutmeg (use ½ a teaspoon of nutmeg

0.333333 cup sugar

Sea Salt (use ½ a teaspoon of sea salt)

Sugar (use 1 cup)

Cinnamon (use 1 tablespoon)

Powdered milk (use 2 tablespoons)

2 piece of egg (use egg yolk)

INSTRUCTIONS

1) Except for powdered milk, cinnamon, ½ cup of sugar and a piece of egg,

2) Put all other items into a mixer and mix into a dough.

3) Put into worm bowl, and set aside in warm place for the dough to rise.

4) When the dough rises, place on the counter and roll out with a rolling pin, and roll till it is 1-inch thickness.

5) Cut into smaller pieces and mold into balls, leave to rise again

6) Use round cutter to make desired wholes

7) Preheat fryer

8) Place dough into the Fry Basket.

9) Break an egg, remove the egg white and use the yolk, mix the yolk and two tablespoons of milk to make an egg wash

10) Brush the doughnuts with egg wash.

11) Slide basket into the fryer and set the fryer to cook at 310 degrees for 15 minutes.

12) Periodically turn the doughnuts to ensure even cooking.

13) When the timer beeps, dish and serve.

Air Fryer Doughnut Bread Pudding

COOKING ITEMS

1½ cup of whipping cream

4 pieces of eggs

Cinnamon (1 teaspoon)

0.75 cup sweet cherries, frozen

1/2 cup of raisin

1/4 cup of sugar

1/2 cup of chocolate baking chips

INSTRUCTIONS

1) Break eggs into bowl remove egg white and use the yolks

2) Put egg yolks, cherries, cream, baking chips and rising into a mixer and mix

3) Add the rest of the cooking items and pour into the Baking Pan. Place foil over the dish.

4) Place the Baking Pan into the Fry Basket

5) Place basket in the fryer

6) Set cooking time to 60 minutes at 310 degrees.

7) When cooked, wait for the meal to cool off, and then serve.

Air Fryer Peach Crisp

COOKING ITEMS

4 cup sliced peaches, frozen

Sugar (3 tablespoons)

White flour (2 tablespoons)

Sugar (use 2 teaspoons)

A quarter cup of white flour

0.333333 cup oats, dry rolled

Unsalted (2 tablespoons)

Cinnamon 1 teaspoon

Chopped pecans, 1 tablespoon

INSTRUCTIONS

1) Put peaches, 3 Tablespoons of sugar, 2 tablespoons of flour and 1 teaspoon of cinnamon in a bowl, mix and pour into the Baking Pan.

2) Place the baking Pan into the Fryer Basket.

3) Set fryer to cook for 20 minutes at 300 degrees.

4) Give the peaches a stir, after 10 minutes.

5) In a bowl mix the rest of the cooking items to make the crisp topping.

6) When the timer beeps, remove the Fry Basket and pour the crisp topping.

7) Place the Fry Basket fryer and set to cook for 10 minutes at 310 degrees.

8) When the timer beeps, let cool for 15 minutes.

9) Serve with your favorite ice cream.

Air Fryer Cheesecake

COOKING ITEMS

Cream cheese (1 pound)

2 piece of eggs

Vanilla extracts (use ½ a teaspoon)

1 cup honey graham cracker crumbs

Sugar (use ½ a cup)

2 tablespoon of unsalted butter

INSTRUCTIONS

1) Cut a circle out of a piece of parchment paper and Place it on the Baking Pan.

2) Mix the butter with graham cracker crust together in a bowl and press into the Baking Pan.

3) Place the Baking Pan in the Fry Basket and scroll to the Roast Icon.

4) Press the Power Button & adjust cooking time to 4 minutes at 350 degrees.

5) Blend cream cheese in a mixer, add sugar, add one egg at a time, add vanilla and mix well until creamy.

6) Remove the Fry Basket from the fryer and pour the cheese mixture on top of the graham cracker crust.

7) Place the cheesecake back into the Air Fryer.

8) Scroll to the Bake Icon and set fryer to cook for 15 minutes at 310 degrees.

9) Set aside for 2-3 hours before serving.

Air Fryer Cherry Pie

COOKING ITEMS

Can cherry pie filling (21 ounces)

Pre-made pie crusts, refrigerated

1 piece of egg, (use egg yolk)

Tablespoon milk

INSTRUCTIONS

1) Place pie crust on the Pie Pan and press. Poke the dough with a fork

2) Place the Pie Pan in the Fry Basket

3) Place fryer in the basket

4) Set cooking time to 5 minutes at 310 degrees F.

5) When the timer beeps, remove the Fry Basket and carefully remove the Pie Pan.

6) Remove the excess dough hanging over the Pie Pan. Pour the can of cherry filling into the pie crust.

7) Roll the last crust out and cut it into 3/4 inch strips.

8) Place the strips going one way across the top and the opposite way across to make a lattice.

9) Mix the egg yolk and the milk and brush the pie with the egg wash.

10) Place the Pie Pan into the Fry Basket and slide into the fryer, set fryer to cook for 15 minutes at 310 degrees F.

11) When timer beeps, set aside, and let cool, then serve with any ice cream of your choice.

Air Fryer Hash Brown Recipe

COOKING ITEMS

4 pieces of potatoes, (shredded and sliced)

Corn flour (2 tablespoons)

Chili flakes (use 2 teaspoons)

Garlic powder (use 1 teaspoon)

Onion Powder (use 1 teaspoon)

Vegetable Oil (use 1 tablespoon)

Ground Pepper

Salt

INSTRUCTIONS

1) Peel potatoes, shred and soak in water.

2) Put 1 tablespoon of vegetable oil in a sauté pan, add shredded potatoes and sauté till its lightly cooked

3) Transfer potatoes to a clean bowl and set aside, add corn flour, salt, pepper, garlic and onion powder and chili flakes and mix.

4) Spread the mixture over a plate and pat it firmly with your fingers.

5) Then refrigerate it for 20 minutes

6) Preheat air fryer to 180C

7) Divide refrigerated potatoes into 2 into equal parts with a knife

8) Brush the basket with olive oil

9) Place the hash brown pieces in the basket, slide basket into the fryer and set to fry for 15 minutes at 180C

10) Check the items after 7 minutes and flip to ensure that it is evenly cooked

11) Dish it hot with ketchup

12) Serve and enjoy

The End